# BEAUTIFUL BROWS

# BEAUTIFUL BROWS

The Ultimate Guide to Styling, Shaping,
and Maintaining Your Eyebrows

## NANCY PARKER
~ and Nancy Kalish

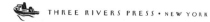

THREE RIVERS PRESS • NEW YORK

Published by Three Rivers Press, New York, New York.
Member of the Crown Publishing Group.

Random House, Inc.
New York, Toronto, London, Sydney, Auckland
www.randomhouse.com

Three Rivers Press is a registered trademark
and the Three Rivers Press colophon is a trademark
of Random House, Inc.

Design by Karen Minster

Celebrity photos courtesy of Photofest New York.

Printed in the United States of America

Library of Congress Cataloging-in-Publication Data
Parker, Nancy.
    Beautiful brows / Nancy Parker and Nancy Kalish.
    (pbk.)
    1. Eyebrows.  2. Beauty, Personal.
    I. Kalish, Nancy.  II. Title.
RL87.P36 2000
646.7'042—dc21    00–030219

ISBN 0-609-80670-X

10  9  8  7  6

# ACKNOWLEDGMENTS

This book would not have been possible without the generous support and encouragement of a number of people. Unknown to me before this project began, Nancy Kalish has been the best partner I could ever have hoped for. As you, reader, are about to see, she's a gifted writer, able to take my sometimes fuzzy thoughts and express them in a clear and fun way. And she's more—always positive, extremely knowledgeable about beauty, able to see different perspectives, and, now, a good friend. I thank Sarah Silbert at Crown Publishing for having the foresight in putting together our team, for ongoing guidance throughout, and for her editorial expertise as our work neared completion. The encouragement of my children, Teri and Michael, and my father, Neil Thompson, has meant a great deal to me. And I thank my best friend and husband, Doug Parker, for his support and all the laughter I'll ever need.

NANCY PARKER
Eyebrowz Designs Inc.

It was an amazing privilege and pleasure to work with Nancy Parker. She is the ultimate eyebrow expert and a wonderful collaborator, always enthusiastic and encouraging, and able to patiently explain even the toughest concepts. It was truly a match made in writing heaven. Thanks to Sarah Silbert at Crown for putting us together and laboring so tirelessly with us to make the book work. I dedicate this book to my beautiful daughter, Allison, who has the best brows.

NANCY KALISH

# CONTENTS

# INTRODUCTION
## Brow Power

It's said that the eyes are the windows of the soul. But the truth is, the eyebrows are. They're the ones that really express your emotions best. (Imagine trying to look surprised or angry without your brows!)

The right brows can be an incredible beauty asset, while the wrong ones can spoil the look of an otherwise pretty face. Many women overlook the humble eyebrow. Big beauty mistake! The reason: Well-shaped brows balance the rest of the face, bringing your best features into focus and downplaying flaws. In fact, changing your brow shape can change the way people perceive you, giving you a more sexy, smart, or confident look—without even switching lipsticks. Just take a look at the photos on pages 10 and 11.

Still not convinced of brow power? The next time you're in a restaurant or another public place, do the brow test. Take a good look at the face of every truly gorgeous woman there and you'll notice something amazing. While they may or may not have big eyes or

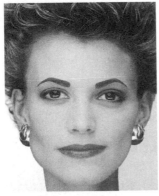

Soft-angled brow

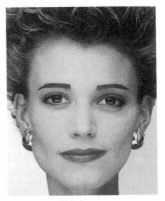

Flat brow

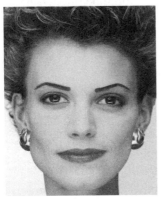

Curved brow

high cheekbones or full lips, there's one thing they are certain to have in common: beautiful brows. And, chances are, they weren't born with them.

You don't have to be, either. While you may need surgery to get the perfect nose or chin, the perfect brows are just a few plucks and a little brow pencil or brow powder away. This is true even if you've never tried to shape your brows before and they're running wild, or you've

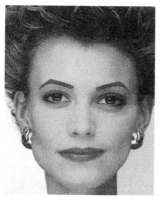
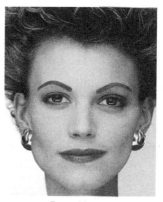

Angled brow                   Round brow

tried too hard and tweezed them into oblivion. This book will show you how to pick the most flattering brow shape for your unique face, and then achieve that shape using a variety of different methods. And we'll blast some annoying brow myths that you may have bought into. For example: No, your brow shape doesn't have to follow your natural brow line (that's like saying your hairstyle has to follow the natural flow of your hair). And, yes, you can pluck the hairs growing above the top of your brow (why would you want to be hairy there?).

After you've gotten your brows into a great basic shape, you can try one of our classic looks for a special night or just for fun—without removing one additional hair. With this book, you have all the brow know-how you need in your hands, not to mention a new power to look your very best every single day. Happy plucking!

# PART ONE

## The Best Brow Formula:

Choosing the Right Shape for You

What's the first tool makeup artists always pull out of their kits to use on models and movie stars? Tweezers!

The reason: The pros know that a pair of perfectly shaped eyebrows can do more for your face than almost any cosmetic. In fact, by correctly shaping and coloring your brows, you can make your eyes appear larger, your face appear slimmer and more shapely, show off your best features, and minimize flaws. You can even mimic the effects of plastic surgery. (Don't you dare get that eye-lift until you see what a little brow shaping can do!) Best of all, the right brow will make you look stylish and well-groomed every single day. And you won't need a makeup artist, because we're going to show you exactly how to do it yourself.

## ANATOMY OF AN EYEBROW

Before we begin, you need to know your brow anatomy so we're all speaking the same beauty language.

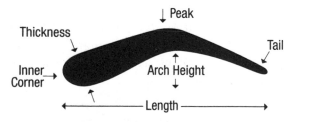

↓ Peak

Thickness

Tail

Inner Corner

↑ Arch Height ↓

← Length →

## THE FIVE BASIC BROWS

There are five basic brow shapes, with dozens of variations. Each one will give you a totally different look–and actually change the appearance of your other features (see the photos on pages 10 and 11).

**Round:** This shape softens the face, literally adding roundness and helping to tone down sharp features, such as a pointed chin.

**Angled:** The high, sharp peak draws onlookers' eyes upward, giving a youthful appearance. The peak creates a strong brow that works well with other strong features such as a square jaw. It can also help slim a round or diamond face. But take care not to angle your brow *too* sharply or highly. It looks horribly fake.

**Soft Angled:** Similar to above, but with a softer and subtler peak, giving the face a more feminine look.

**Curved:** This flattering shape projects a feeling of confidence and professionalism. It works especially well on a square or oval face.

**Flat:** Perfect for those with long faces. The horizontal lines of this brow make the face appear shorter and more oval.

While all these brow shapes may look intriguing, you have to choose yours carefully–or the results can be disastrous. For example, an angled, highly arched brow can help make a round face appear more oval, but a round brow can turn that same face into a beach ball. And the angled, highly arched brow that's so attractive on a round face will make a long face look even longer.

You can certainly have fun with different brow looks, such as those in Part Three. But to determine the very best brow shape for you–the one you'll want to wear every day–you need to thoroughly analyze your face and individual features before you even go *near* a pair of tweezers. This is much easier than it sounds. We'll show you how in four simple steps.

**STEP ONE:**     Find Your Face Shape
**STEP TWO:**     Figure Out Your Signature Features
**STEP THREE:**   Determine Your Best Brow Strength
**STEP FOUR:**    Put It All Together

**Stop!** We know you're tempted to skip these steps and start tweezing. But don't jump ahead just yet. If you want to look truly great (and we know you do), all of the following info is *essential*. And we promise, we'll keep it quick and painless (if only we could say the same thing about tweezing!).

## STEP ONE: Find Your Face Shape

Have you ever really thought about the shape of your face? Probably not. But knowing whether it's round, long, square, heart-shaped, diamond-shaped, oval, or some combination is extremely important. Why? The shape of your face not only dictates which brow shapes will look good on you, but also which hairstyle and makeup decisions you should make. (Have you ever noticed how a high forehead on a long face is helped by bangs? Or how a square jaw can be softened by a shoulder-length mane?)

No one shape is better than another. The trick is just to find out as much as you can about your own face, and then use that information to enhance it.

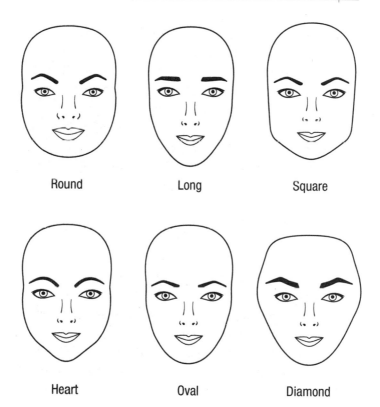

Round · Long · Square

Heart · Oval · Diamond

## What's Your True Face Shape?

Pull your hair back from your face and remove all makeup; then take a good look in the mirror. Though your face may not *exactly* match one of the descriptions below, it will probably come pretty close. If not, ask yourself which shape it is *predominantly* and follow the recommendations for that. Here are some clues to help you figure out your true shape: If...

. . . your face is almost as wide as it is long, and widest at the cheeks, it's probably **round.**

. . . your forehead, cheekbones, and jawline are all about the same width, it's probably **long.**

. . . your forehead, cheekbones, and jawline are all about the same width *and* your jaw is square, it's probably **square.**

. . . your forehead is wider than your chin, your cheekbones are the same width as your forehead, and your face tapers to a pointed chin, it's probably **heart-shaped.**

. . . your face is widest at the cheekbones or temple, your forehead is short and narrow, your face tapers to a pointed chin, and your features are angular, it's probably **diamond-shaped** (fairly rare).

. . . your forehead is slightly wider than your chin, your cheekbones are prominent, and your face tapers to a narrow oval, it's probably **oval.**

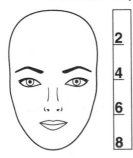

## Still Not Sure? Take This Simple Face Shape Test

**A.** Using a ruler, measure the length of your face from crown to chin.

**B.** Divide the answer by 3.

**C.** Measure the distance from the bottom of your nose to the bottom of your chin.

**Results:** If the answer to B is greater than the answer to C, your face is probably long or square. If the answer to B is less than C, chances are your face is round or possibly diamond. If B and C are equal (or close), your face is most likely oval or heart-shaped. It's probably oval if you have a round chin, heart-shaped if you have a pointed chin.

## So What Brow Is Best (and Worst) for You?

Choosing the correct brow shape for your face can make or break your whole look. So we've outlined a few definite (you-don't-want-to-mess-with-them) rules. And though this book is supposed to stick to brows, we couldn't resist throwing in a few extra hair and makeup tips. You can have great brows and still blow it with a hairstyle that's all wrong for your type of face. We just couldn't let that happen!

## Round Face

**Best Brow:** Angled with a high arch and a short tail. This shape makes the face look longer and slimmer. But don't angle your brow too steeply or it will look misplaced and just draw attention to the roundness of your face.

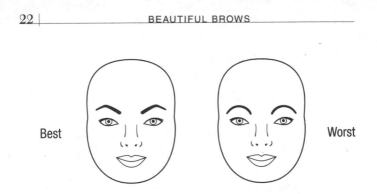

Best                                                      Worst

**Worst Brow:** Round, a shape that echoes the shape of the face and makes it appear even rounder.

**Other Must-Know Info: Hair:** Use hair to slim your face by wearing a style that has some height at the crown and not too much volume at the sides. Skip a chin-length bob, which makes the face look rounder. Hair should either fall above the chin or below it. **Makeup:** Don't forget to accentuate cheekbones with just a touch of blush. Apply it on your cheekbone, starting directly below the inner corner of the eye and slanting upward toward the temple. This will help further thin your face. Another essential beauty aid: a sexy shade of lipstick (don't be afraid to try a red that's right for your complexion). Luscious lips draw attention away from wide cheeks and make you look very kissable.

## Long Face

**Best Brow:** Flat and horizontal, which makes the eye look side to side rather than up and down, making the face appear more oval.

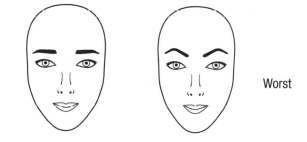

Best                                                                Worst

**Worst Brow:** An angled brow with a high arch and a short tail will exaggerate the length of your face.

**Other Must-Know Info: Hair:** Seek out styles with volume on the sides, especially around the cheeks and ears. Bangs will also help bring better proportion to a long face, making it seem shorter, while a deep side part will widen your cheekbones. Avoid middle parts, especially with straight hair, which only emphasize your face's narrowness. **Makeup:** Blush is a big helper here. The best way for you to sweep it on is horizontally, starting at the *outer* corner of the eye. Some makeup artists also advise putting a dab of blush on the chin to shorten it. While this can be effective, be careful. Too much will make your chin look like it's one big zit! Something else to think about: High neck-lines are very flattering to this face shape, but plung-ing ones are not. If you want to show off your cleavage, consider a neckline that's cut in a wide V rather than a deep, narrow one.

## Square Face

**Best Brow:** Angled with a sharp peak OR curved with a sharp peak to focus attention away from a square jaw and balance the face.

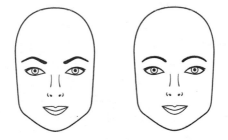

Best                                                                 Worst

**Worst Brow:** There is no brow shape that will make the jaw look more square. But a delicate, rounded shape won't balance a strong jaw.

**Other Must-Know Info: Hair:** Soft styles, especially those with layers and wisps around the face, are by far the most flattering. The real no-nos: super-straight styles and blunt, chin-length bobs—both of which accentuate a strong jaw. **Makeup:** Try a dab of light foundation or concealer on your chin to highlight it and make your jaw seem less square. Use a shade only *slightly* lighter than the rest of your face and blend well.

## Heart-Shaped Face
**Best Brow:** Rounded to "soften" the point of the chin.

Best 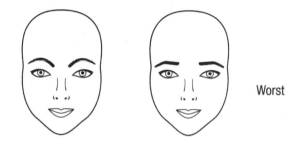 Worst

**Worst Brow:** A flat, horizontal brow, which does nothing to counterbalance the point of the chin. The result: The whole equilibrium of the face is thrown off.

**Other Must-Know Info: Hair:** Go for styles with some fullness at the bottom, such as a chin-length bob or another style that adds some curls around the chin, which will help round out your face. **Makeup:** Take some time to find the perfect shade of lipstick for your complexion. Once you do, don't leave home without it. Along with the right brow, it will help you balance your face and complete your look.

## Diamond-Shaped Face

**Best Brow:** An angled brow or a curved brow with a peak will "narrow" your wide cheekbones and temple, and give your face another focal point. A round brow is another good choice because it will bring softness to an angular face.

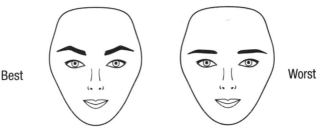

Best                                    Worst

**Worst Brow:** A flat brow will make this face shape appear unflatteringly short. By drawing the viewer's eyes side to side, this brow also makes a wide face appear even wider.

**Other Must-Know Info: Hair:** Diamonds look wonderful in styles that add some fullness around the bottom of the face. A classic rounded bob with bangs that falls to the chin is a perfect example of a style that balances both a narrow forehead and chin, making the face look more oval. Stay away from any style that starts to curve outward at the cheekbones. **Makeup:** Avoid deep shades of blush, which will just emphasize your wide cheekbones, and don't overdo the application. Instead, play up your eyes and mouth equally to help balance your face.

## Oval Face

**Best Brow:** Any shape that enhances your features, like the soft angled brow shown. Since your face is already oval, brows play no role in making it appear more so.

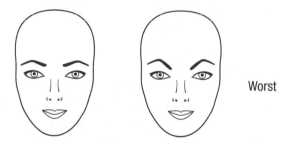

Best                                                              Worst

**Worst Brow:** One that's not groomed properly—or at all. Or—and this is a major error—a brow that's too highly arched, giving the face a look of perpetual surprise or anger.

**Other Must-Know Info: Hair:** You can wear almost any style. The one caveat: Don't hide that beautiful face shape. For example, heavy bangs that cover your forehead will camouflage the symmetry of your face. **Makeup:** Apply blush carefully, or it can make your face seem wider or narrower. The color should start on the cheekbone directly below the center of your eye and sweep upward toward the temple.

## STEP TWO: Figure Out Your Signature Features

Before you start plucking away, remember that your face shape isn't the only factor in determining the best brow shape for you. Your features, especially the strong ones, also come into play.

Often, we think of strong features, such as a prominent chin or large nose, as undesirable because they stand out. But the truth is, a strong feature simply needs to be counteracted by *another* strong feature in order to make the face look balanced. That's where eyebrows come to the rescue.

It's a law of nature: When people look at your face, their eyes automatically fall on the most prominent feature simply because it's the first thing they really see. But correctly shaped eyebrows can literally *redirect* the onlooker to see the *entire* face instead of focusing on just one part of it. That's why beauty experts often say that the right eyebrows can "open up the face."

Perhaps even more important, a good set of brows will draw attention to the eyes (often our best feature) and away from those features we're less crazy about. Sometimes women use heavy makeup to play up their eyes, but this can look artificial. When you use your brows instead, people will think you have bigger eyes and a more balanced face *naturally.* They'll think you've done something new with your hair or makeup, but they won't be able to put their fingers on it. (Don't you just love those "You look great . . . what have you done to yourself?" moments?!)

## Finding the Right Balance

In order to establish what eyebrow shape will best help balance your features, you need to figure out which features really need balancing. Do you have delicate or strong facial features? Some women have features that are all about the same size, with no individual feature that stands out. If this is really true about you, you can skip right to Step Three. Many women, however, have one or more features that do stand out, such as the eyes, nose, lips, or chin. To determine which of yours need "brow balancing," it helps to do an overall feature assessment.

If there was ever a time to be completely truthful with yourself about how you look, it's now. Remember: There's truly no such thing as bad features, only a bad job at assessing them. Having trouble? Get a trusted friend to help you. You can promise to do the same for her. Then you can use the how-to's in the next part of the book to do brow makeovers on each other.

Ready? Now pull your hair back from your face once more and take a good honest look in the mirror. Where are your eyes drawn first? Your nose? Your lips? Your chin? That's probably the feature others focus on, too. And, as a result, they could be "missing" the rest of your face. For example, a prominent nose can easily distract onlookers from your smaller, but lovely, eyes. Here's how to deal with this and other strong features.

## Large Eyes

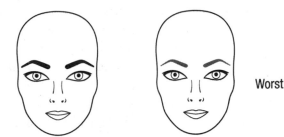

Best　　　　　　　　　　　　　　　　　　　　Worst

Big eyes are certainly a big beauty asset. But they definitely need strong brows to accompany them. If your brows are light and delicate, your eyes can look *too* large, and take over your face. This is especially true if you accentuate your eyes even more with makeup. To make your brows appear stronger, deepen the color or add thickness, perhaps below your brow line since the closer your brows are to your eyes, the stronger they will appear. And you can help your brows do their job by wearing a vibrant lip color. This will further balance your face with a strong feature at the bottom. It's important to make the most of your eyes—but not at the expense of the rest of your face.

## Almond Eyes

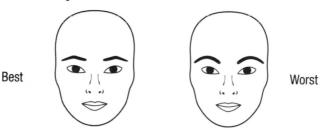

Best

Worst

The cat-like beauty of this eye shape can be emphasized by the right brow. Whereas a rounded brow will make the eyes look rounder, an angled brow will draw attention to the upper part of the face and emphasize the lovely shape of the eye. Asian women with almond eyes often have other delicate features as well, and care must be taken that the brow doesn't overpower them. Thin brows can be a strong black. But if your brows are thicker, you might want to try a slightly lighter shade to balance delicate features.

## Prominent Nose

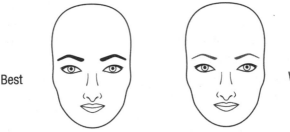

Best                                        Worst

If your nose is currently the focus of your face, you can use your eyebrows to divert that attention. For example, flat brows or any shape that's too light and delicate will do nothing to distract from a large nose. But highly arched brows literally point away from the nose, and you can add to this effect by making them deeply colored and thick as well. This not only helps balance your face, but also makes your eyes more prominent, drawing people in. The overall effect can be stunning. For example, Barbra Streisand certainly has a large nose, but her strong, angled brows draw attention up and away from it. Of course, everyone still notices that Streisand has a large nose. There's no way, short of plastic surgery, to make it petite. But her brows (along with some well-applied eye makeup) help make her nose balance harmoniously with the rest of her face. And such a transformation is possible for us large-nosed mortals as well. Just take a look at what the right eyebrows can accomplish in the best-and-worst on the opposite page.

## High Cheekbones

Although professional models come in all different face shapes, they do seem to have one feature in common: cheekbones to die for. High cheekbones add a beautiful, slimming angularity to any face. Of course, you can fake them with blush. But if you really have 'em, we say flaunt 'em. Surprisingly, one of the best ways to do that is with a brow that echoes their shape with a high angled arch and a tail that points down to draw attention to—what else?!—those cheekbones.

## Pointed Chin or Large Lips

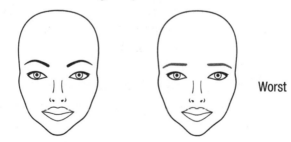

Best                                                Worst

These features both have the same effect: They draw attention away from the eyes and toward the lower part of the face. Again, balance is the goal—and it's easy to accomplish with the right set of brows.

Rounded eyebrows can provide a soft contrast to a pointed chin, for example, as shown in the illustration on page 33. The same brow shape can be used to balance large lips as well.

## Glasses: Don't Make a Spectacle of Yourself

If you wear them, you know: Putting on your glasses can change the way your whole face looks, and not always for the better. They act like the strongest facial feature there is, sometimes fighting against the rest—and winning. You may sometimes feel like tossing them (if only you didn't have to see!). But don't head for the wastebasket or order contacts just yet.

Picking out a pair of glasses can seem so hit or miss, but we've found a way to take the "miss" out of it. It turns out that the best pair of specs is the one with a frame that follows the line of your brow. Once you find the right brow shape for you, it will help guide you to the right frame.

One no-break rule: Stay away from glasses that copy your face shape. Round frames on a round face will make it look (you guessed it!) even rounder, while square frames on a square face will make it look like one big block. Instead, just as with brows, think about counterbalancing your face shape. For example, if your face shape is:

**Round:** Try angular styles that are no wider than the widest part of your face. Square frames with a curved edge can also be flattering.

**Long:** Round, oval, or square frames are best, especially those with a colored top bar, which creates a strong horizontal line, widening the face.

**Square:** Choose curved styles that are no wider than the widest part of the face. Frames with more color at the outer than inner edges also work well. Whatever glasses you pick, they will be most flattering if their shape appears more vertical than horizontal.

**Heart:** Aviator or butterfly frames do a good job of balancing this shape. Slightly curved rectangular frames can look great, too—as long as they're not wider than your forehead.

**Diamond:** Gently curved or square frames are a good counterpoint to the angles of this face shape, especially if they are heaviest on top. Look for styles that have straight sides or sides that angle outward at the bottom. Be sure to stay away from styles that are wider than your cheekbones—you don't want to add even more width there.

**Oval:** You can wear just about any style, as long as it's in proportion to your face. But be sure that the frames are not too large or much wider than your cheekbones.

## STEP THREE: Determine Your Best Brow Strength

We've said it before, but it's worth saying again: The goal is to achieve a balance with your face shape and features. To accomplish this, it often helps to pair like with like. Strong, prominent features call for a strong brow. Delicate features call for a light brow. Of course, playing around with different strengths is the best way to find out what works for you.

There are three things that affect brow strength:

**1. Proximity to the eye: The closer the brow is to the eye, the stronger it will appear.** The brow and eye work together to create and define the eye area. If they are too close together, the result is a tight, closed-in look as seen in the illustrations on the opposite page. But you can open up the area by plucking excess hairs from underneath the brow line.

**2. Thickness: The thicker the brow, the stronger it will appear.** This is pretty self-evident, but some women still fail to take it into consideration. It's easy

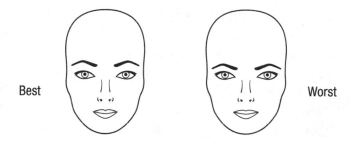

Best                                                    Worst

for a thick brow to look top heavy, especially if you don't have large eyes to balance it. If that's true for you, a little thinning can do wonders (see "Bushy, Coarse, or Curly Brows" in Part Two for the best technique).

**3. Color: The darker the brow, the stronger it will appear.** Making your brows lighter or darker affects the overall balance between your features–and the first time you see yourself with a new brow color, it can throw you for a loop. It's like trying on a bright red lipstick that's very flattering but is still a little shocking when you see yourself in the mirror. (See "Choosing the Correct Color" in Part Two for our tips.) So give yourself some time to get used to a new color before you decide it's not for you.

## STEP FOUR: Put It All Together

By now you probably know more about your face shape and your features and how your eyebrows can work with them (or against them) than you ever thought you would.

Still, if these concepts are new to you, it can be difficult to see just how to apply them to your own unique face. To help out, we've done brow make-overs on five regular people (no professional models allowed!), each with a different face shape and signature features, so you can see for yourself the incredible effect the right brow can have. Also check out the classic looks in Part Three to see how the right brows helped solve certain stars' beauty problems.

Finally, look for eyebrow inspiration in the faces all around you. Examine whether a person's brow shape really goes with her face and why or why not. If a woman looks great, chances are that one of the reasons is that her brows really work for her. Find women with faces like yours and do mental brow makeovers on them. It's fun and you can learn a lot from their mistakes and successes before you start shaping your own brows.

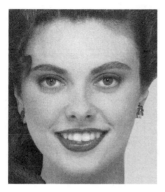

**Before**

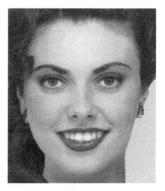

**After**
Removing hair from below
the brow line creates a
lighter, more feminine look.

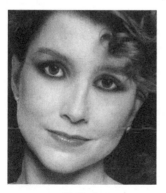

**Before**

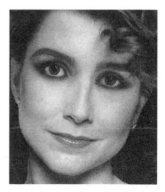

**After**
Making the brows stronger
with brow powder brings
balance to heavy eye makeup.

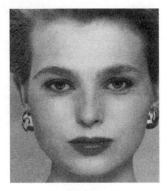

**Before**

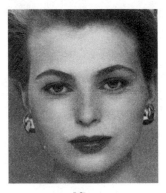

**After**
Reshaping the brow
with a sharper peak gives
the eye area a lift.

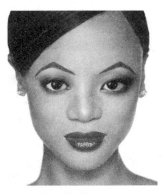

Adding a sharp peak
emphasizes the
cat-like beauty of the
almond eye shape.

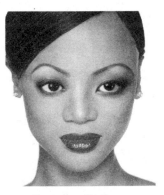

Rounding the brow
will make the eye appear
rounder as well.

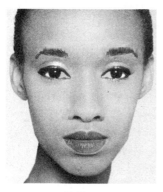

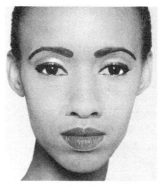

**Before**

**After**

Creating a flat brow makes
a long face look shorter
while the downward curve
of the inner corners
balances larger lips.

# PART TWO

## Define and Conquer:

How to Shape, Color, and
Re-create Your Brows

Whether you're an old pro at plucking or a brow virgin (never been tweezed!), this section contains all the how-to's you'll need to shape your brows just the way you want them, and then keep them that way. Whatever your previous eyebrow experience, the tips and techniques that follow should be part of your beauty repertoire. Once you master a few tricks, you'll see how simple it is to have beautiful brows every day—and you'll marvel at the incredible difference they can make to your face.

But before we get started, we want to bust some common myths that you may have bought into. Not only are they untrue, they could be standing between you and beautiful brows.

**Myth #1: Your eyebrow shape has to follow your natural brow line.** As we mentioned in the introduction, that's like saying your hairstyle has to follow the natural flow of your hair—complete nonsense. A lot of ugly brows out there are the result of this natural-is-better belief. What's important is to find the shape that's most flattering to your face. If it follows your brow line, great. If not, it's time to learn what actresses and models have known all along: There's nothing wrong with making your brows longer, more highly arched, thicker, or a different color. The only thing you have to lose is bad brows.

**Myth #2: Your eyebrows are the frame for your face.** It's because of meaningless beauty babble like this that eyebrows often get overlooked and ignored. A frame doesn't have the ability to make or break a piece of art the way brows do when it comes to your face. You must think of your brows as an important feature, right up there with your eyes and lips–not just as two things stuck up at the top. That's the only way you'll give them enough emphasis in your beauty routine to bring out their best.

**Myth #3: You should never pluck the hairs above your brows.** This is one of those rules that are held up as beauty gospel but don't actually make much sense. Why would you want to be hair-free below your brow but not above it? It is true that brow hair is more fragile than other facial hair and grows back more slowly. So you want to be judicious about removing it–from above, below, or around the brow. It's also true that removing the hairs below the brow will probably do more to improve your brows than removing hairs from above. But if you've carefully planned out your brow look by following the instructions in this book and decided that those hairs should go, we give you permission to do it.

**Myth #4: Using makeup to enlarge or change the shape of your brows will make them look too fake.** Okay, no one wants to do a Joan Crawford and end up with scary black caterpillars on their forehead. But if you use a light hand, it's easy to use brow powder and pencil to create a totally natural-looking brow—even if you're adding a long brow tail or an inner corner where none was before. And yes, even if you are artistically challenged. It's a little like using blush or lipstick for the first time. You just need practice. (See "Finishing Touches: Using Brow Pencil, Powder, and Gel," later in this part, for some helpful tips.) Even if you're not making any major changes to your brows, filling in any blank spots and enhancing them with some powder or pencil will make them look smoother and more polished. People probably won't be able to figure out exactly what you've done to your face; they'll just think you look fabulous.

## THE TOOLS OF THE TRADE

It's always easier to do a good job if you have the right equipment, and shaping eyebrows is no exception. Here's what's worth investing in.

## A Brow Brush or Comb

Just like head hair, some brow hair can be hard to manage (yes, your brows can have a bad-hair day!). Enter the brow brush. This handy little tool will help you groom and style your brows every morning. Brushing also helps remove dirt and dead skin particles that get trapped under brow hairs. The best brush shape depends on your type of brow hair. If you have long brow hairs that won't lie the way you want, a mascara wand-style brush will give you more control than a straight brush. If your brow hair is very thick or so coarse it appears almost brittle, the hairs probably won't bend around a wand-style brush. In that case, your best bet is a brow comb. In a pinch, an old toothbrush can be reborn as a brow brush, provided the bristles are still strong and the toothpaste is long gone.

## A White Pencil

This pencil (available at the drugstore) makes it easy to mark exactly which hairs you need to get rid of—think of it as Wite-Out for your brows. Use it to sketch the outline of the shape you want (even easier if you use stencils—see next page), and white out the hairs you want to remove. You can also use concealer applied with a cotton swab or a small brush. If your brows are so light that you can't see the white pencil, use a black eyelining pencil instead.

## Eyebrow Stencils (Optional)

Used since ancient Egyptian times, stencils take all the guesswork and stress out of trying a new brow shape. All you do is follow the outline and, voilà! You can see exactly where you need to pluck. Stencils also make it much easier to properly fill in sparse or over-plucked brows with pencil or powder (see "Sparse or Overplucked Brows," later in this part). Perhaps most important, stencils ensure that both brows turn out precisely the same way. After using the stencil on one brow, you simply flip it over to get a mirror image on the other brow. Of course, you can also create great brows without stencils. It just may take more practice to get the shape exactly right. (See Resources, at the end of the book, for more information on my stencil kits and Web site.)

## Eyebrow Pencil

This is another must-have brow tool for many women, although some light-haired women should skip it alto-gether. But for those with medium or dark hair, an eye-brow pencil is great for darkening or coloring brows without adding volume the way that powder does. It provides precise application for filling in blank spots. For the artistically inclined, it can even be used to draw on realistic brow hairs. And since it adds color to both hair and skin, it makes it easy to define the edges of your brows so they look super smooth. Sharpening a brow pencil can be tough, however. The trick is to place the pencil in the fridge overnight or the freezer for ten minutes to harden it. Or buy a mechanical pencil, which requires no sharpening at all.

Brow pencils are available in a wide range of colors, and the shade you choose will affect how strong your brow appears and the way it balances with your other features. (For more information on picking the right color, see "Choosing the Correct Color," later in this part.)

But even though many beauty books and magazine articles say you must use pencil to define your brows properly, the truth is brow pencils don't work for everyone. On some women–especially those with blond, strawberry blond, and graying hair–they can look too harsh. If you're one of those, the secret is to forget pencils and use brow powder alone. It stays on just as well as pencil but will give you the more realistic results you've been looking for. What a relief! You'll wonder why no one ever told you this before.

## Eyebrow Powder and Brush

Simple to apply quickly and evenly, colored brow powder creates a soft, natural-looking eyebrow. Like pencil, powder can also be used to create a nice smooth edge. Powder also adds volume to the brows–

a real plus if yours are sparse or overplucked. In fact, it can be used to essentially "paint" on a pair of brows if there aren't any there at all. But because of this, brow powder is best on light and/or sparse brows. It can be too much on top of those that are already dark and/or full. The exception: We've found that powder looks great on African-American women because it beautifully complements dark skin.

Just as with pencil, you need to choose your powder shade carefully. Many people custom-mix more than one color to get the exact right shade.

## Tweezers

Even if you mainly use another method of hair removal, you still need tweezers to remove those annoying stray hairs that seem to pop up overnight. And if you regularly shape your brows by plucking, a really good pair is an absolute must.

Tweezers should be able to firmly grab an individual hair and pull it out easily. Often, badly made or old tweezers don't grip properly. There's nothing more frustrating than finally grabbing hold of a big ol' ugly hair just to have it slip out of your grip as you are getting ready to pull! But when you have a good pair of tweezers that can pluck the little sucker right out . . . ahhh, that's satisfaction. It's like repeatedly missing your golf swing, only to finally connect and hit a hole in one. So if your tweezers aren't doing the job, toss 'em and get a pair that will. Also keep in mind that after a while, the ends of your tweezers may become dull. This means you may need to sharpen or replace them every once in a while. Tweezerman, which makes some of the best pluckers around, offers a lifetime guarantee as well as free sharpening. (See Resources for more information on Tweezerman products and services.)

The next question: Should you go for a slanted, flat, or pointed tip? The truth is, it's really a matter of personal preference. That said, if you have lots of hard-to-grip fine hairs, ingrown hairs, or brow stubble, you may find it easier to use tweezers with a pointed tip. Those with coarse hairs or tweezing novices may find it easier to go with a slanted or flat pair. Do avoid tweezers with scissorslike or other gimmicky grips—they are generally harder to control.

The last consideration is comfort. It's especially important for a professional makeup artist or stylist to use a pair that doesn't cause hand strain. But this is true for the rest of us as well. If your tweezers are uncomfortable, don't suffer—get another pair.

## Nail Scissors

These are good for trimming those hairs that extend beyond the outline of your brow. A nail clipper will also work—just remember to clip only one hair at a time.

## Brow Control Substances

There are a number of products that help style brows that resist cooperating on their own. Brow gel, which is applied with a mascara-like wand and comes in clear or colored versions, not only sets the hairs in place but also moisturizes them, making them more pliable and easier to work with. If your brow hair is sparse, you might want to consider a colored gel which can help give the appearance of more volume. Using a little hairspray on your brow bush will also keep willful hairs in their assigned spots.

## GOOD RIDDANCE: The Best (and Worst) Hair Removal Methods

In the war against excess eyebrow hair, there are many weapons. Some are easier and more effective than others—and a few are downright dangerous. So you must choose carefully. Just because you use a method on your legs, bikini area, or even another part of your face doesn't mean you should use it on your brows. One reason: Eyebrow hair is very different from the hair on the rest of your body.

~ Eyebrow hair is *much less* influenced by hormonal changes than the rest of your body hair.

~ Eyebrow hair grows *very slowly*–four times more slowly than scalp hair. If you overpluck your brows, it can take three to eight weeks for them to grow back in.

~ Eyebrow follicles are sensitive to injury, such as waxing, plucking, or electrolysis. Repeated injury may cause follicles to shrink (creating thinner, finer hairs), sprout hairs growing in a different direction, or stop producing hairs altogether. So think first: If you permanently damage your follicles, you will be left with the same look forever.

There are three basic ways to remove brow hair (or any other hair on your body):

**1.** Break hair at or near the skin surface (shaving, trimming, depilatories).

**2.** Remove the whole hair from the root (tweezing, waxing, sugaring, threading).

**3.** Apply heat to damage the hair follicle underneath the skin, removing hair and perhaps preventing further growth (electrolysis, laser hair removal).

Hair

Follicle

Now that you understand brow biology, here's a rundown of all your removal options and our recommendations.

## Just Say No

**Depilatories:** The FDA warns against using a chemical hair dissolver on eyebrows because of the possibility of its dripping into—and permanently damaging—your eyes. In addition, leave a depilatory on too long and it starts to remove your *skin* (truth!), something to keep in mind if you use this product on any other part of your body as well. **Pluses:** None. **Minuses:** You're risking blindness.

## Proceed with Caution

**Shaving:** Many women swear by shaving to shape their brows. You can even buy mini razors specially made for the eyebrow area (see Resources). **Pluses:** Quick, inexpensive, painless (unless you get a nick), and doesn't affect the color or texture of regrowth. **Minuses:** Grows in quicker than other methods. And because shaving creates a flat top to hair, regrowth may appear more coarse and bristly at first (it eventually returns to softness). This method works best if your skin and hair are both light or both dark, since the inevitable stubble that occurs once your brows start growing back won't show as much. Brunette beauties with light skin, however, beware: Shaving your brows is a mistake unless you're prepared to do it each and every day. Otherwise, you will end up with slow-growing stubble that's very visible to everyone– but too short to pluck out with tweezers.

**Trimming:** It's a great idea to *slightly* trim hairs that hang over the edges of your brows (see "Don't Forget to Trim," later in this part). But cutting hairs all the way down to the skin's surface is generally a no-no for the same reasons given for shaving, above.

**Threading:** This method is practiced in Asia and Europe, and is gaining popularity elsewhere. A piece of cotton thread is rolled over the area of unwanted hair, which causes the hairs to twist around it. The technician then pulls on the thread, which, in turn, pulls the hairs caught around it out by the root. Threading should be done only by a highly skilled professional. **Pluses:** Regrowth takes three to eight weeks, and hair may grow back lighter in color and texture. **Minuses:** Expensive because it must be done at a salon; some pain.

**Electrolysis:** Electrolysis uses an electric current to damage the follicle so the hair doesn't grow back.

**Pluses:** Although more painful than waxing, it lasts a lot longer. It takes several visits to be sure the electrologist has zapped all the hairs in their growing phase (the period when they are most vulnerable), but eventually the results are permanent. A topical anesthetic, EMLA, is available by prescription for electrolysis done elsewhere on the face. EMLA is not recommended for use on the brows because of their proximity to the eyes, but you don't really need it anyway. Just grit your teeth and think about how you'll soon be rid of all those pesky strays. To find a licensed or board-certified electrologist, see Resources. **Minuses:** This method can be permanent, so it's best limited to hairs that obviously grow way beyond the brow line. For this purpose–as well as cleaning up those annoying strays on your upper lip or chin–it's excellent.

**Laser Hair Removal:** Lasers are hot, literally. Like electrolysis, this popular new kid on the hair removal block uses heat to permanently damage the hair-producing follicle. A directed laser beam passes through the skin and heats only the follicle. **Pluses:** It's quick and not too painful–it feels like you're being lightly snapped with a rubber band, and your skin may look sunburned afterward. **Minuses:** It's really expensive and must be done by a highly skilled professional, preferably an M.D. Laser proponents say that hair removal is permanent or near-permanent, making this method better for hairy legs than hairy brows—unless it's to zap only those hairs you're sure you'll never need.

## Go for It!

**Tweezing:** It may be low-tech, but tweezing is our favorite form of brow hair removal. **Pluses:** It's easy to do, precise, effective, convenient, and cheap. Once you've got your brows in shape (see "How to Tweeze Like a Pro," later in this part), all you need to do is a minute or two of maintenance every few days to keep them looking great. What could be easier? **Minuses:** It can be so addictive, it's easy to overpluck. In fact, some people even suffer from trichotillomania, a psychological disorder that compels them to pluck and pluck until there's nothing left.

**Waxing and Sugaring:** There are three types of waxing: hot, warm, and cold (see "How to Wax Like a Pro," later in this part). They all work basically the same way. Wax is applied to the brow, the wax sticks to the hairs, and then it's ripped off *fast* like a Band-Aid being removed (ouch!). Sugaring is a very similar method, supposedly first practiced in ancient Egypt. It uses a warm, gooey, and, yes, sugary paste, which sticks to hair and is then removed. You can find myriad home waxing and sugaring kits at your local drugstore, or you can have the process done at a salon. **Pluses:** Regrowth takes three to eight weeks, and hair may grow back lighter in color and texture. Inexpensive, if done at home. Good for areas where you want to remove a lot of hair. While waxing and sugaring do hurt a bit, the pain is blessedly brief. In addition, sugaring has some advantages over waxing: It sticks only to hair (unlike wax, which sticks to both hair *and* skin). This means a little less pain during the process, and almost no irritation afterward. **Minuses:** Hair needs to be at least a quarter-inch long to be removed (especially if it's coarse), so you'll need to let it grow in between sessions. Waxing and sugaring are not as precise as tweezing; you'll probably still have to pluck a few hairs here and there afterward. Sometimes waxing can also cause ingrown hairs. Finally, waxing should not be done at all if you've been using certain medications or skin creams (see complete list in "How to Wax Like a Pro," later in this part).

## EYEBROWS FOR DUMMIES: Brow Shaping 101

For many women, there's a lot of anxiety about shaping their eyebrows. They're afraid they'll do it wrong.

Well, it's true that you can do it wrong. But it's also not that hard to do it right. We'll show you how to start with some basic brow cleanup, then progress to precise shaping by either waxing or tweezing. If you need some moral support (and some help making sure both brows are even), get a trusted friend to assist you. Then do the same for her.

One word of caution, however. The temptation is to take your tweezers and start plucking away. But we advise you do just the opposite. As we've mentioned, once removed, brow hair grows back extremely slowly, if at all. So, after you've done some initial cleanup and shaping to create a good everyday look, stop plucking and live with your brows for a week or so. Then, before you go any further, use the techniques in Part Three (which involve no *additional* hair removal) to test-drive that high arch you've always wanted *before* you actually pluck it into place– and perhaps make it permanent.

And since a variety of looks are so easy to fake with some powder and pencil, you may not want to make any of them permanent at all. That will give you the flexibility to try out one of our fabulous classic looks for a fun night out or whenever the mood strikes you.

# ARCH ENEMIES:
## The Most Common Brow Problems

Sometimes the beauty gods seem to conspire against you and give you brows that are harder than average to manage. Here are some of the most common problems and how to solve them without stress.

## Bushy, Coarse, or Curly Brows

If your brows are very thick and wild, it's probably wise to do a little extra taming before you start to shape them (see "Basic Brow Cleanup"). Here's how: Brush your brow hair straight up. Trim any hairs that extend *way* above the brow line. **Caution:** Do not trim these hairs even with the top of your brow line or they will be too short when they are brushed back into place—and even harder to control. They should still extend about three-eighths of an inch beyond the top of the brow. You can always prune them more later.

Next, thin out the center of the brow a bit. Use a white pencil (or dark pencil if your hair is light) and mark a dot every quarter inch along the center line of your brow. Then tweeze out just a hair or two at each dot. If possible, pick the coarsest hairs (or those that have lost their color) to pluck. Don't worry about creating an arch at this point, and don't be tempted to overpluck. Step back and reevaluate your progress in the mirror frequently. The goal is simply to thin your brows without creating any holes. Then you will be ready to do more reshaping, if necessary.

If your brow hair is coarse or curly, it can be brittle and hard to manage. The solution: Treat your brow hair like your head hair and use conditioner in the shower to soften your brows and make them easier to style. Or try slightly wetting your brows before styling. After shaping and styling your brows, keep them in place with brow gel and the right brow brush or comb (see "The Tools of the Trade," at the beginning of this part). If that doesn't work, try a *tiny* dab of extra-strength hair gel and gently work it through the hairs with a stiff brow brush.

## Sparse or Overplucked Brows

Perhaps your brows have always been naturally sparse. Or maybe you went a little crazy with your tweezers and now you're left with brows that barely show at all or that have major gaps. If you're not in the habit of overplucking, your brows may grow in again, although it can take several weeks. Or the condition may be permanent. Either way, however, it's not hopeless.

In fact, in some ways it can be easier to shape a sparse brow. The quickest and least stressful way to do it is with a stencil (again, see "The Tools of the Trade"). You can also do it freehand, but unless you are really artistic, your brows may end up looking asymmetrical

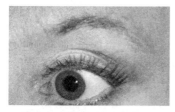

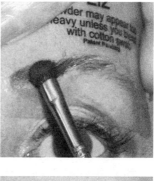

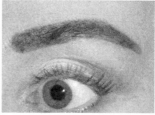

and fake. Use Part One of the book to figure out the most flattering brow shape for your face. Then position your chosen stencil in the place where your brow should be and fill in with either brow pencil (using short, hairlike strokes) or brow powder (which adds much-needed volume). You may also want to try pencil with powder over it to achieve the most natural look. This method will not only create a brow where there was barely one before, but it will also cover any messy stubble as your hairs grow in. Ironically, you still have to tweeze any hairs that grow outside your brow line.

## Complete Brow Hair Loss

Some conditions, such as alopecia areata, thyroid problems, certain autoimmune diseases, or undergoing chemotherapy, can cause you to lose some or all of your brow hair. If this is the case, you can use stencils and eyebrow powder to create a natural-looking brow. The key is to choose the right stencil (see "The Tools of the Trade") and position it correctly (see "The Pencil Trick: Where to Start, Arch, and End," on the next page). Then fill it in with brow powder, not pencil, which can give the brow that drawn-on look you want to avoid. For more tips on using brow powder properly, see "Finishing Touches," later in this part).

## A Sagging Brow Line

Unfortunately, gravity is a fact of life. Unless you spend your days standing on your head, your brows will migrate south as you get older, along with the rest of your body. A sagging brow area can make it difficult to create a brow shape that's true and flattering. But there is a remedy. Simply hold the skin up and taut while applying your brow pencil or powder. When you let go, the brow will fall back into position and look natural. Also: Consider adding a higher peak to your brows. While you should choose the best brow shape for your face shape and features, adding a higher peak will give some much-needed lift to your brow line.

# BASIC BROW CLEANUP

There's an old saying that we've discovered applies to eyebrows: Sometimes you can't see the forest for the trees. Translation: Before you can start shaping your brows, you need to get rid of all the stray hairs that obviously fall completely outside the brow line and clutter your eye area.

The easiest way to do this preliminary cleanup is with tweezers (see "How to Tweeze Like a Pro" later in the part). You can also have it done by an electrologist. But beware of removing too much hair at this stage. You just want to zap the little strays that are growing way below the brow bone (close to your eyelid), across the bridge of your nose, or otherwise far outside any brow shape you could possibly want. **Note: Do not remove any hairs above the tail or outer corner of your brow—yet.** You may later find that you want to "lift" the tail so it runs more horizontally and will need the hair there. If not, you can always remove it later.

## The Pencil Trick: Where to Start, Arch, and End

This is also the time to do what pros call "the Old Pencil Trick," a simple method of figuring out the exact spots where your brows should start, arch, and end. Those spots will be the same no matter what brow shape you choose. You can either remove the hairs that grow outside those boundaries now as part of your basic cleanup, or later when you do more precise brow shaping.

Traditionally, this technique has been done with a regular lead pencil. But if you do it with a makeup pencil that contrasts with your hair and use it to mark the right spots with a dot, it will be much easier to find them when you start to shape your brows.

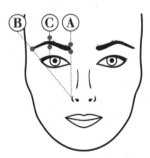

**A.** Take a white pencil (if your hair is medium to dark) or dark eye pencil (if your hair is light) and position it in a straight line, running from the outside of your nostril up to the inner corner of your eye. Use the pencil to mark two dots where it crosses the brow, one at the top inner corner and one at the bottom inner corner. This is where your brow should start.

**B.** Next, angle the pencil so it runs from the outside of your nostril to the outer corner of your eye. Use the pencil to mark one dot where it crosses the brow. This is where your brow should end.

**C.** Finally, line the pencil up so it runs straight up and down along the outside of your iris. Use the pencil to mark two dots where it crosses the brow, one on the bottom edge of the brow and one on the top edge. This should be the brow's highest point, the top of the arch. However, if the brow shape you want is fairly flat (the most flattering for a long face), the arch can look nice a little farther out (see Audrey Hepburn's brow in Part Three). Make one dot on the top edge if you want a sharp peak, two dots if you want a more rounded peak. Then connect the dots. Repeat steps A, B, and C with your other eye.

## But What If . . .

This trick works well if your eyes are spaced perfectly (approximately one eye-width apart). But what if your eyes are wider set? Or closer together? In addition, a wide nose can throw you off. Here's how to deal with those special circumstances.

## Special Circumstance #1: Close-Set Eyes

If you have close-set eyes, you just need to use a little imagination. The goal is to create the illusion that your eyes are spaced more widely—and it's not that hard. All you have to do is *pretend* that you have more space between your eyes and then use the pencil trick. So, for example, if your eyes are closely spaced, move them one eye-width apart in your imagination to find the correct inner and outer brow corners. That means

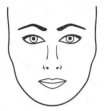 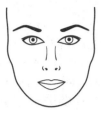

If your eyes are close-set, using the regular formula will make them look closer.

But, if you start your brow's inner corner farther from your nose, your eyes will look less close-set.

that your brows should start farther from the inner corner of your eye, as in the diagram above right. As you can see, this makes the eyes look wider. **Note:** Don't be tempted to start your brows *too* far apart, or it will just accentuate the closeness of your eyes. So do this test first: Use a concealer or white pencil to cover up the inner brow hairs you're planning to remove, and take a good look in the mirror before you actually do the deed.

## Special Circumstance #2: Wide-Set Eyes

For widely spaced eyes, simply "move" your eyes slightly closer (approximately one eye width) in your imagination to find the correct inner and outer corners. The result: Your brows will be closer together than your eyes are, and, as you can see in the illustration on the opposite page, this will make your eyes seem more closely spaced. So if you've been plucking the inner

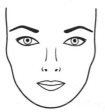

| If your eyes are wide-set, using the regular formula will make them look wider. | But, if you start your brow's inner corner closer to your nose, your eyes will look less wide-set. |

corners according to the old formula, cease and desist. And if your brows don't naturally start as closely as you'd like, consider extending the inner corners with pencil or powder.

## Special Circumstance #3: A Broad Nose

If your nose is wide and you do the pencil trick, the inner corner of your brows may end up too far apart. If that's the case, just pretend your nose is not all that wide. Don't be afraid to align the pencil with the *middle* of your nostril to find the most flattering inner corner. But before you pluck, be sure to cover the hairs you plan to remove with concealer or white pencil to see if the new starting point really suits you.

## CONSIDER YOUR INNER CORNER

You've probably never thought much about the inner corner of your brow, and yet the shape of it can communicate a lot about your character and make a big difference in your look. There are five basic inner corners that you can combine with any brow shape you desire. You should think about which will work best for you before you start shaping your brows, and tweeze or wax accordingly.

 **Oval:** The most common inner corner, this shape has a pleasing roundness that will soften your look.

 **Sleek:** This slimmer version of the oval comes to more of a point at the end. The result: a sexy, catlike effect.

 **Block:** This corner makes a strong statement and works especially well with a very thick brow. But it is the very opposite of overgrown. Its clean edges give it a very crisp, assertive look.

 **Teardrop:** The button end of this corner has a very feminine, almost cute appeal while still looking intelligent.

**Tufted:** Brushed up and wispy, this corner gives
the brow a natural—yet still well-groomed—look.
You don't need to remove any hair to achieve it.
Simply brush up the inner corners when you're
shaping and styling the rest of the brow.

## DON'T FORGET TO TRIM

Some women
are so caught
up in tweezing or waxing
that the simple act of trimming—and the terrific
way it can take care of straggly brow hairs—is forgot-
ten. Others are afraid that using scissors on their
brows breaks an important beauty rule. Well, it's just
not so. In fact, all some women need to do is trim in
order to achieve a polished look. So we wholeheart-
edly give you permission to prune your brows . . .
a little.

Trimming is used on those hairs that are in the
right place but are so long that they stick out above or
below the outline of your brow, creating an unkempt
look. Most of the time, it's a good idea to trim *before*
you tweeze or wax, since it makes it easier to see the

brow line. The trick is to trim just enough so that the edges appear nice and smooth. Cut too much, however, and you'll go from looking shaggy to spiky, which is no more attractive.

To trim the body of the brow, brush the hairs up. Then use cuticle or nail scissors (or even a nail clipper) to trim a tiny bit off of the longest hairs, one hair at a time. **Caution: Do not cut hairs down to the top line of the brow—they** will be way too short when you brush them down again. Brow hair should be left at least several millimeters *above* the brow line. Trim a few hairs, then brush your brows back into shape and assess them. Then trim a bit more if necessary, and reevaluate again. Before you take off too much, remember that brow hairs grow *very* slowly.

Another place you may want to trim is the tail of your brow, where the hairs grow downward on some women. If this is the case, brush the hairs at the tail *down*, then carefully trim them just slightly longer than the bottom of your brow. Brush back into place.

Spotting errant hairs and learning exactly how much to trim them will become easier with practice. Just keep at it and take it slow.

# HOW TO TWEEZE LIKE A PRO

When you're working with your eyebrows, every hair counts. That's why tweezing, which removes only one hair at a time, is the perfect way to shape your brows. Some women get their brows tweezed at a salon (a good idea if you're still uncertain of the best shape for your face). But as long as you work slowly and thoughtfully, there's no reason why you can't pluck them just as well at home. In fact, you'll probably find you're just great at shaping your brows with tweezers the very first time you try, especially if you use stencils. And after you've gotten your brows into shape, it takes only a minute or two every week or so to get rid of any hairs that dare to grow outside the line. (For our tips on what type of tweezers to use, see "The Tools of the Trade," earlier in this part.)

One warning: Don't let yourself get too pluck-happy. Many women make the mistake of overtweezing. This is especially common when you're trying to achieve a smooth edge to your brows. It's like trying to even out a home haircut. You take a little off one side, only to find you need to take a little off the other side to even it up. And then before you know it, you're almost bald! Our advice: Don't worry about your edges now. At the end, we'll show you how to smooth them out without tweezing too much.

## Pre-Plucking Prep

**1.** The best time to pluck is after a hot shower. Or remove your makeup and place a hot facecloth on your brows to soften hair and open pores. The worst time to tweeze? If you already have your makeup on (plucking will make your eyes water). You should tweeze at least thirty minutes before applying makeup, and it's best to do it a whole day in advance if you have a special event and don't want to take the risk of having a ring of pinkish skin around your brows.

**2.** Do not apply any face cream or moisturizer before plucking. It may make your tweezers slip.

**3.** Work in good light. Daylight or an illuminated mirror will allow you to see every hair.

**4.** Most important: Map out a clear strategy. Know exactly what shape you're going for before you even pick up your tweezers. If you haven't already done so, the first step is to use the pencil trick described earlier to place dots in the spots where your brows should start, arch, and end.

If you are using stencils, it's easy from here. As the photos show, all you need to do is place the stencil over your brow, making sure the inner and outer corners line up with the correct dots on your brow. Then use a white pencil to outline the shape and remove the stencil. We've taken an overgrown brow and given it a softly angled shape. Of course, the procedure is the same no matter what shape you desire.

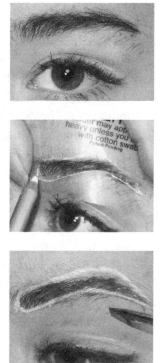

If you are not using stencils, carefully draw the outlines of the brows with the white pencil. Use the dots you've just made and the illustration of the brow shape you desire (see "The Five Basic Brows" in Part One) as guides. If that's too tough, use the white pencil to draw only the *bottom* edge of the brow. Plucking the hairs from the bottom will have the most effect anyway.

**5.** Then do this pre-tweeze test: White out all the hairs below the line with your pencil or some concealer—and take a really good look in the mirror. Is the arch too high, or not high enough? Make adjustments as necessary and check again.

## Ready, Set, Tweeze

**6.** Starting with the bottom of your brow, tweeze one hair at a time. Since brow hair can grow sideways, it's important to pluck one by one and check where the root of each hair is so you can be sure you won't create a bald spot. Then grip each hair individually as close to the root as possible and pull gently in the direction it grows–don't yank. If this is your first tweeze in a while, remove one row of hair from the bottom of the brow at a time. Then step back and evaluate. When you're happy, do the bottom of the other brow the same way.

**7.** Now move on to the top of your first brow. There's no rule against removing hair from the top of your brow. Some people worry that it's easy to take off too much there, but we say: not if you pluck carefully. Some people also worry that if you pluck, the brow hair will grow back thicker. Remember: Eyebrow follicles are easily damaged by things such as plucking, so hair is likely to grow back more finely, if anything. Start with the hairs that are obviously above the outline of the stencil or above the line you've drawn in your mind of where you want your brows to be. If you have doubts, stop there. Think about it for a few days. You can always pluck more later if you want to.

**8.** If plucking is painful, apply pressure with your fingers after each tweeze. You can also try numbing your skin with a topical toothache medicine, such as Anbesol. But frankly, it smells so yucky, we'd rather suffer. After tweezing, wash off the white pencil and any concealer.

**9.** If using a stencil, place it back on and fill in any small gaps with eyebrow powder or a sharp eyebrow pencil, using small, feathery, hairlike strokes. Even if you're not 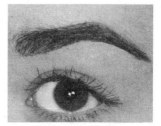 using a stencil, you can fill in any gaps the same way. (See "Finishing Touches," at the end of this part, for more tips.)

## HOW TO WAX LIKE A PRO

We think waxing and its sister, sugaring, are wonderful, quick ways to do basic shaping on your brows. You can get your eyebrows waxed at a salon or use one of the home kits available at any drugstore. If you're worried that you might not be able to handle shaping your brows this way, it's a good idea to have a professional do it the first time. Then you'll know just where to apply the wax for future touch-ups.

Since waxing removes large amounts of hair at one time, it may be less painful than tweezing hairs out one at a time. But you will still have to do some plucking to catch any strays. **Caution: Users of Retin-A, Renova, Accutane, and corticosteroids such as hydrocortisone, prednisone, Kenalog, and Elocon should not use a wax hair remover at all.**

These medications thin the skin and can result in skin being pulled off along with the wax. Creams containing alphahydroxy and betahydroxy acids may cause the same reaction. A waiting period of six months after discontinuing most of these drugs and creams is recommended before attempting to wax. Accutane users are advised to wait seven years (yep, you read right!). Other medications may cause skin thinning, so check with your doctor before waxing. And never wax on sunburned or broken skin or you risk the same effect.

If you do decide to wax, go slow and take the time to prepare your brows properly—especially if this is your first time. You need to place the wax in *precisely the same spots* on both brows in order get symmetrical results. Using an eyebrow stencil will make the process a lot easier and exact, but you can also draw on the desired shape freehand.

## Choosing the Right Kit

There are many different kinds of home waxing and sugaring kits on drugstore shelves. Some contain premade wax strips. Others feature a small jar or tube of wax or sugar paste, with or without clothlike disposable strips to press down on top of the paste, making it easier to remove. Some types of wax or sugaring solutions also need to be heated in the microwave or a bowl of warm water. Be sure to choose a kit with *water-soluble* wax or sugar paste so you can easily wash away any mistakes you make. Most of the kits are inexpensive, so it pays to experiment until you find one you like. Kits with premade wax strips are good for those using stencils because you can draw on the shape of the brow you want and then cut it out. But those that come with jars of paste are most economical because there is less waste. We go over the basic procedure for waxing and sugaring below, as well as give you some extra tips that will ensure you end up with the brow shape you want. But always be sure to follow the manufacturer's directions carefully.

## Pre-Wax Prep

Waxing is best done at night or another time when you can give the stripped areas a chance to recover before putting on makeup. And remember: Just as with tweezing, it's better to wax too little than too much. You can always tweeze out any extra hairs at the end— a lot better than having to wait until a bald spot grows back in.

Following is a never-before-waxed brow, whose owner wants it to be a soft-angled brow. We'll take you step-by-step through the transformation, which is the same no matter what new brow shape you want to create.

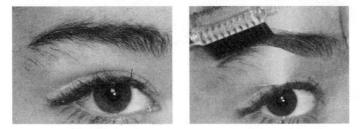

**1.** Gather everything you will need: your kit, an eyebrow brush, and a white pencil or concealer to outline brow shape. If using stencils, you'll also need transparent tape, a ballpoint pen, and a craft knife (available at arts and crafts stores) or a small pair of sharp scissors. Read the kit's instructions carefully.

**2.** Wash thoroughly to remove all cosmetics and creams and dry well. If it's hot weather, dust the area with talcum powder to absorb perspiration.

**3.** Use the pencil trick to be sure where your brow should begin, arch, and end, and mark the spots with dots.

**4. No Stencil:** Brush the eyebrows hairs roughly into the desired shape.

**Stencil:** Place the stencil on your brow, lining the corners up with the dots. Brush hairs through stencil, guiding them toward the outer corner of your brow and into the desired shape.

**5. No Stencil:** Use the dots to help you carefully draw the outlines of the brows you want with the

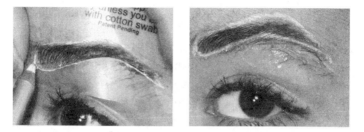

white pencil. Or, if you prefer, draw only the bottom of the brow. Removing the hairs from the bottom of the brow will have the most effect anyway. Repeat with other brow. Check carefully for symmetry. Note: If you're doing this freehand, it's especially important to draw on both brows *before* you begin waxing so that you are sure they will be even and the same shape. If you don't like what you see, wash it off and try it again. To be extra sure, white out the hairs you'll be removing with your pencil or some concealer so you can see what you'll look like after waxing.

**Stencil:** Outline desired shape in white pencil. Remove stencil.

## Doing the Deed

**6.** If using a wax or sugar paste, carefully apply the paste to the areas outside the white pencil outline, usually in the direction of hair growth (but check manufacturer's directions). Do the bottom of both brows first, then the tops; this will make it easier to make sure you're waxing evenly. (See special directions below for using premade wax strips with stencils.)

**Caution: If you make a mistake and place the wax or strip incorrectly, do *not* pull it off.** Most wax and sugar pastes are water soluble. Simply wet the area down until the strip slides off, wash off any residue, dry completely, and try again. **If you get wax on your eyelashes, don't panic and start pulling.** Keep your eye closed and gently wash the wax off your lashes.

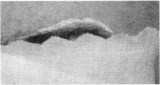

**7.** If your kit comes with it, apply a clothlike disposable strip and press it down.

**8.** Holding the skin taut with one hand, let 'er rip! Pull the strip off *very* quickly in the *opposite* direction of hair growth. Do it too slowly and the wax (and your hair) will remain behind.

**9.** Use your fingers to put pressure on the area to relieve pain and any redness that might occur. Many kits include some kind of soothing lotion or cream to apply afterward, some with topical analgesics such as Benzocaine. If you tend to get ingrown hairs, swab the area with an antiseptic (exfoliate the area regularly with a gentle scrub to prevent them).

**10.** After redness has subsided, use a pencil to outline the edges and fill in blank spots for a smooth, polished look. (See "Finishing Touches," below, for more tips.)

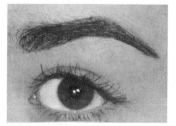

## Using Stencils with Wax Strips

If you are using stencils and premade wax strips, you can create a precise pattern for waxing your brows. Here's how:

**1.** Place a wax strip specifically sized for brows on a cutting board. Center the stencil on it and tape it down.

**2.** Using a ballpoint pen and, pressing firmly, outline the brow shape. Remove the stencil.

**3.** Using a craft knife or sharp scissors (the knife is a lot easier), very carefully cut out the entire *inside only* of the brow shape. Do not cut through the outside edge of the strip. You should be left with a perfectly brow-shaped hole in the middle of the wax strip, as if you had just used a brow-shaped cookie cutter on it. You can toss the piece you just removed. You can also wax only the bottom part of your brow this way by tracing only the bottom edge of the stencil onto the wax strip.

**4.** Working super slowly, carefully peel the backing off of the wax strip (it's *very* fragile and tears easily). Line up the brow-shaped hole along the white outlines you've drawn on your brow. Press down. Then proceed with step 8, above.

## FINISHING TOUCHES:
## Using Brow Pencil, Powder, and Gel

Okay, the painful part is over. You've removed all the stray hairs and gotten your brows into good shape. Now you just need to add a few finishing touches to make them look really great.

### Choosing the Correct Color

The general rule of thumb is that your brows should be two shades lighter than your hair. But the exact opposite is true for blondes and those with light hair: Brows should be two shades darker than hair color. African-American and Hispanic women generally find dark brown brows to be the most flattering, while Asian women look best in a soft black color.

But the rules can—and sometimes should—be broken. Some blondes look great in black brows (think Marilyn Monroe). Brunettes with auburn highlights can look stunning with some auburn added to their brows with brow powder or pencil. And makeup artists sometimes like to bleach the brows of dark-haired models really light for a barely there look that can be very chic. You might want to try "lightening" your own brows with some foundation, yellow shadow, or colored mascara, however, before you reach for the bleach (though you can always put the color back with some brow powder or pencil).

Brow bleaching must be done extremely carefully. First of all, there's the whole issue of using such a strong chemical so near your eyes. Personally, we'd rather fake light brows than risk it. If you decide to do it anyway, use a very small amount of facial bleach (available at the drugstore) and keep it as far away from your eyes as possible. Bleach works *fast*. Test to see the color every few moments by wiping away one of the corners. As soon as you achieve the shade you want, wipe it off, then rinse the area thoroughly. Since bleach affects the protein structure of the hair, it can make your brows brittle. Prevent this by dabbing on some hair conditioner after you're all done.

Don't be afraid to play with color to achieve different brow strengths. For instance, if you like your brows thick, you can still lighten your look by lightening their color a bit. Also, keep in mind that just like the hairs on your head, the hairs in your brows are several different shades. To re-create this natural effect, try combining different colors (blond and light brown, for example) and different mediums (pencil and powder). But if this is too time consuming, here are the right shades that will do the quick trick.

| IF YOUR HAIR IS | TRY |
| --- | --- |
| Blond | Blond powder, blond or taupe pencil |
| Light brown, strawberry blond, or red | Light brown powder, blond or taupe pencil |
| Auburn | Auburn powder, taupe pencil |
| Medium brown | Medium brown powder, brunette pencil |
| Dark brown or black *and/or* you're African American or Hispanic | Dark brown powder, dark brown pencil |
| Black *and* you're of Asian descent | Soft black powder, black pencil |
| Gray | Soft charcoal powder, slate pencil |
| Purple, yellow, or other fun colors | Jet black (looks cool at raves and no one will dare ask for your ID) |

Even if you love it, resist the urge to make your new shade permanent. Tinting or dyeing eyebrows is dangerous, and the FDA has issued warnings against it. One reads that the FDA "prohibits the marketing of hair dyes for eyelash and eyebrow tinting [because] this practice has been known to cause severe eye injuries and even blindness." Many women have also had horrible allergic reactions to the dye, which also colors the skin underneath the brow temporarily.

Getting a darker brow tattooed on is also a bad idea—even if you've suffered irreversible eyebrow loss from alopecia or another medical condition (see "Sparse or Overplucked Brows," earlier in this part, for other solutions). If you tattoo them and you're not happy with the results, too bad—it's probably permanent. Your best bet: Stick to brow powders and pencils, which will do the job just as well or better.

## Filling In the Blanks

Most brows have little bald spots. You can use either brow pencil or brow powder to fill them in (or even some eye shadow in a pinch). As we mentioned earlier, brow pencil works well for some women, but others—especially those with light hair—may find it too harsh. In that case, brow powder alone is a good choice. Powder is also your best bet if your brows are sparse and you need to fill in large areas—or want to increase brow thickness or arch height for a special night out—because it creates a natural, full look. But for this reason, women with already full brows should probably use pencil instead.

**To apply brow pencil:** Use a sharp pencil to fill in blanks with light, hairlike strokes in the same direction that the hair is growing. Afterward, always go over the area with a clean, stiff brow brush to soften the look and make it more realistic.

**To apply brow powder:** Use a small hard brush with a flat, angled tip, made especially for this purpose. This shape makes it easier to control and apply powder just where you want it. Dip just the tip of the brush into the brow powder and then tap it once or twice against the container to get rid of any extra. Fill in blank spots with light strokes (you can always go over your brows again, if necessary). If you're trying to draw on large parts of your brow (such as the tail), balance the hand holding the brush against your face to steady it. Work slowly and add a little powder to one brow, then to the other, stepping back often from the mirror to make sure both brows are even. Also: Make sure you know exactly where the tail should end. If you don't, see "The Pencil Trick: Where to Start, Arch, and End," earlier in this part.

Afterward, always use a cotton swab to "erase" any excess powder and soften the overall look. A good-quality brow powder should stay on all day and not come off in the rain or if you sweat. To be absolutely sure, look for one that is water-resistant.

## Solving Pencil and Powder Problems

Achieving a truly natural look can take practice. Here's how to fix some common mistakes.

**If your brows look too dark,** use a cotton swab to gently remove some of the color (use a light touch so it doesn't smear all over). Then use a stiff brow brush to soften it some more. You can also pat pressed facial powder lightly over your brows. If the color is still too dark, switch from brow powder to pencil, which might give you exactly the look you want.

**If your brows look too light or not natural enough,** try switching from pencil to brow powder, which has a much softer look.

**If your brows look crooked or you've made another mistake,** use a cotton swab dipped in a *non-oily* makeup remover to gently erase the mistake (an oily remover will make it impossible to reapply makeup). Pat the area dry, then start again.

**If the color won't adhere,** try applying a very tiny amount of moisturizer to the area. This will give the powder or pencil a better surface to stick to.

## Smoothing the Edges

Don't skip this step: It's the key to creating a polished, finished look. Just like outlining your lips gives them definition, so does outlining your brows. Using a pencil that matches the color of your brow, lightly outline the entire brow along the *edge* of the hairs–not on the skin above, or your brow will look like it's been outlined. And remember, easy does it! It doesn't take much to create a smooth edge, and too much penciling will make it look fake.

If you are creating a brand-new brow area (say, a long dramatic tail or a square inner corner) where no hair currently exists, you'll need to make the edge look defined yet believable. You can achieve that by using either a stencil and powder, or by using a brow pencil to create the new edge and then filling in the blank spots with powder. Either way, be sure to tone down any hard lines by lightly going over them with a cotton swab and then a brow brush.

## Keeping the Hairs in Place

Brow gel or mousse fixatives should be applied last. They are either clear or colored, and can add a little shine. They keep brow hairs in place and help set your brow pencil and powder. Some come with a mascara-style brush that's easy to use. If yours doesn't, you can use an old toothbrush. Hair gel or hair spray (sprayed on the brush, not on your brows!) can also be used in a pinch. Whatever product you use, do it very sparingly. It only takes a teensy amount to hold brow hairs in place; more may make a gunky mess and force you to start over.

## BROW UPKEEP

Now that your brows are beautiful, we know you want to keep them that way. All you have to do is stay on top of the strays. It's certainly a lot easier than starting the shaping process all over again.

True tweezing junkies don't need any reminders. They don't even need a mirror—they rely on touch. As soon as they feel a bit of stubble, they pull out their tweezers and take action. But even if you're not as brow-obsessed, it's still important to make brow upkeep one of your regular beauty habits. Setting up a maintenance schedule can be as simple as placing a pair of tweezers and a mirror in a drawer by your television. Every week when your favorite show comes on, you can tweeze those strays away during commercials.

Or get in the habit of examining your brows every morning as soon as you get out of the shower, and tweezing if necessary. You'll have two or three hairs to remove at most, and any redness will have subsided by the time you've dried your hair.

We recommend tweezers for maintaining your brows. They are cheap, travel well, and are easy to pull out anywhere, anytime. A magnifying mirror is also a great help for zeroing in on strays while they're still in the stubble stage or if you usually wear glasses.

Even if you don't need to pluck, use a brow brush daily to keep hairs in place and whisk away any dead skin particles. If the skin under your brow hair is dry, use a moisturizer at night. When skin is moist, it's easier for brow powder and pencil to adhere.

Of course, even if you forget to tweeze for a while and your brows grow back in, don't panic. Remember: You shaped them before and you can do it again.

# PART THREE

## Beyond Basic Brows:

Classic Looks to Try for Fun

**Y**ou may think you know your stars, but can you guess which brow belongs to which celebrity? The answers are at the bottom of the page.

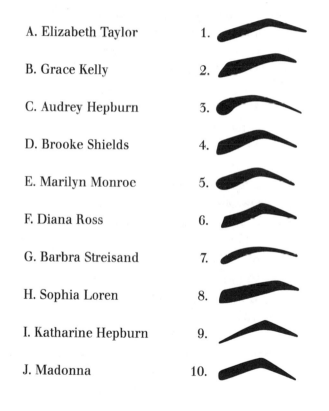

A. Elizabeth Taylor       1.

B. Grace Kelly            2.

C. Audrey Hepburn         3.

D. Brooke Shields         4.

E. Marilyn Monroe         5.

F. Diana Ross             6.

G. Barbra Streisand       7.

H. Sophia Loren           8.

I. Katharine Hepburn      9.

J. Madonna                10.

# TIME FOR A LITTLE FUN

On the following pages, you'll find ten classic looks that epitomize the best in brows. Each has been modeled after a celebrity who exemplified that look. Some, like Audrey Hepburn, are true eyebrow icons, who came up with a totally new shape that they made their signature. Try one if you want to add some pizazz to your everyday eyebrows for a special occasion, or if you just feel like experimenting a little. For example, you can use a new brow look to pump up your sex appeal for a hot date or to project a strong, confident persona at work. Or just try out a bunch of brow looks for the sheer fun of it. (You can find dozens of additional current and classic celebrity brow stencils at www.eyebrowz.com.)

The best part: Once you've plucked or waxed your brows into a flattering everyday shape, you can try out any of these star brows *without any additional plucking.* It's as simple as changing your eye makeup—and can make an even bigger impact. If you use stencils, the transformation will take mere minutes. If you don't have stencils, you'll need to practice a bit. As with everything else concerning eyebrows, it's best to take it slow. Remember the first time you tried to apply eyeliner correctly? After a few tries, you'll be able to get the look you want.

If the look calls for a brow that's thinner than yours,

don't start plucking. Brush your brow hairs down flat, compressing them into a skinnier line. Then gel them into place. For more useful tips, see "Finishing Touches" in Part Two.

What you'll need: brow pencil, brow powder, brow gel, brow brush, and eyebrow stencils (optional). Tip: Always use a sharp eyebrow pencil. Hardening the pencil in the freezer for ten minutes will make it easier to sharpen properly.

## Before You Begin

Start with a well-groomed brow in the most flattering shape for your face (see Part One). Take the time to really study the brow you're copying. Note where it's thickest and thinnest, how high the peak is, how long the tail, and, most important, all the ways in which it differs from the brow you currently have.

Although you can certainly try any of the star brows in this section, you'll have the most success with those geared toward your face shape (we've noted the best matches). Also, remember that the stars on the following pages were made up for the stage and screen, and so their brows are colored very strongly. You may want to copy the shape but tone down the color for a more natural look. Or you may want to play it up and go for the drama. Either way, we say experiment and enjoy all the different looks you can achieve.

## SOPHISTICATED
### As Seen On: Elizabeth Taylor

If we had to pick one perfect brow shape, this would be it. This brow begins, arches, and ends in exactly the right spots, and the smooth edges give it an elegance that never goes out of style (Taylor has worn this basic shape for her entire career). The relative thickness and jet-black color of this brow lend the wearer a look of extra strength and charisma.

 **The Brow:** Soft angled with a high arch and a block corner.

**Best For:** Oval or round face, if you make the tail a bit shorter.

**How to Get It: 1.** Using a brow brush, start at the inner corner and brush the hairs upward and across the brow, guiding them toward your natural peak. Brush the tail hairs down and out toward the outer corner. **2.** Using a brow pencil and the pictures as a guide, extend the inner corner of your brow up and then across to meet your peak. **3.** Carefully create a higher peak, if necessary, with light strokes of your pencil. Round out the peak to avoid a sharp angle. **4.** Draw in the bottom edge, parallel to the top. Fill in blank spots with brow powder. Repeat with other brow. **5.** Use brow pencil to taper the tail of your brow to a point. **6.** To create a smooth edge, outline the whole brow lightly in pencil and gel in place, if necessary. Repeat with other brow.

You can also use stencil inspired by Elizabeth Taylor's brow (see Resources).

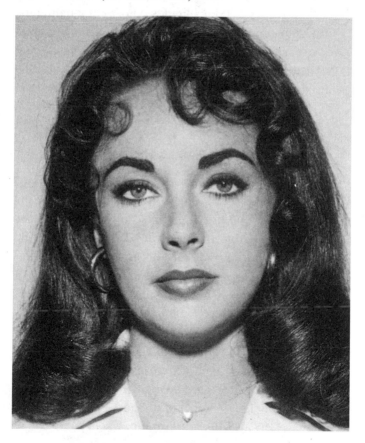

## ELEGANT
### As Seen On: Grace Kelly

This understated brow has a polished, feminine beauty. Though not a thin brow, if it's not made too dark, it works well for blondes who want a light look. But keep in mind that it's too neutral to balance a large nose or other signature features (no wonder it worked so well on Grace Kelly's perfect face!). Instead, this brow will blend in with the rest of your features and quietly enhance them.

 **The Brow:** Soft angled with an oval corner.

**Best For:** Oval face.

**How to Get It: 1.** Using a brow brush, start at the inner corner and brush the hairs upward and across the brow, guiding them toward your natural peak. Brush the tail hairs down and out toward the outer corner. **2.** Using a brow pencil and the pictures as a guide, create an oval shape at the inner corner. **3.** Then starting at the top of the inner corner, extend the top line of the brow up and across to meet your natural peak. **4.** Carefully create a higher peak, if necessary, with light strokes of your pencil. Then round out the peak to avoid a sharp angle. **5.** Draw in the bottom edge, parallel to the top. Fill in blank spots with brow powder. Repeat with other brow. **6.** Using pencil, taper your natural brow tail to a point. Keep in mind that in this case, the tail measures about half the total length of the brow. If yours is too short, extend it. **7.** To create a smooth edge, outline the whole brow lightly in pencil and gel in place, if necessary. Repeat with other brow.

You can also use stencil inspired by Grace Kelly's brow (see Resources).

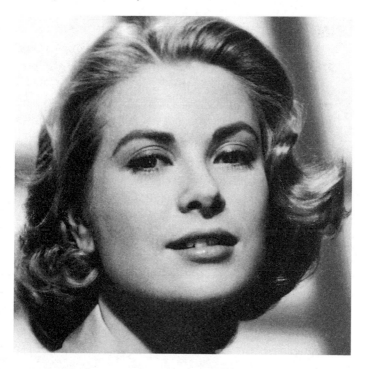

## INNOCENT
### As Seen On: Audrey Hepburn

Hepburn first grew out her thin brows for the role of *Sabrina* in 1954, and they quickly became her signature. At first glance, these big, strong brows may seem too much for a delicate face. But their strength emphasizes the eyes and makes them seem larger. The result is a playful, pixie look that's boyish *and* beautiful.

**The Brow:** Flat with a block corner.

**Best For:** Long face with strong brows.

**How to Get It: 1.** Using a brow pencil and the pictures as a guide, extend the inner corner of your brow up slightly and then across to meet your natural peak. Fill in blank spots with brow powder. If you feel the inner half of your brow isn't thick enough, extend it upward and across a teensy bit more. Repeat with other brow. **2.** Carefully create a higher peak, if necessary. **3.** Thicken the brow tail, bringing it to a short, horizontal point. If your natural brow tail extends downward, don't try to cover it. Instead, thicken it slightly, bringing it to a point, and you'll still get the same look. **4.** To create a smooth edge, outline the whole brow lightly in pencil and gel in place, if necessary. Repeat with other brow.

You can also use stencil inspired by Audrey Hepburn's brow (see Resources).

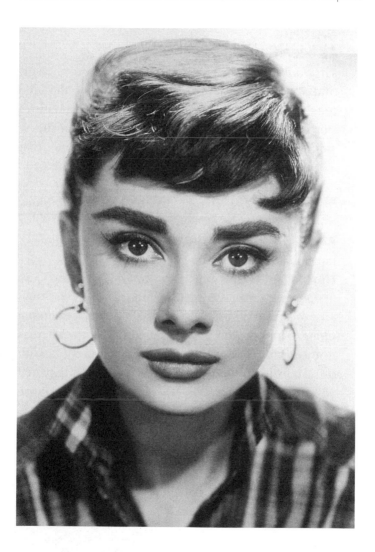

## NATURAL
### As Seen On: Brooke Shields

This look shows that strong brows can be very beautiful. But totally untamed, they're not. While the little tufts at the inner corners provide a lovely natural starting point, the tails have been groomed to a super-smooth edge. If you want an "untouched" look that still has some polish, try this brow shape on for size.

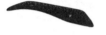 **The Brow:** Flat with a tufted block corner.

**Best For:** Long face with large eyes or a big mane of hair to balance the strong brow.

**How to Get It: 1.** Using a brow brush, brush the hairs at the inner corner straight up to form a tuft. **2.** Using a brow pencil and the pictures as a guide, extend the inner corner of your brow up slightly and then across to meet your natural peak. Fill in blank spots with brow powder. Repeat with other brow. **3.** Using pencil or powder, thicken the brow tail, bringing it to a short, horizontal point. If your natural brow tail extends downward, don't try to cover it. Just thicken it slightly and bring it to a point, and you will still get the same look. **4.** To create a smooth edge, outline the whole brow lightly in pencil and gel in place, if necessary. Repeat with other brow.

You can also use stencil inspired by Brooke Shields's brow (see Resources).

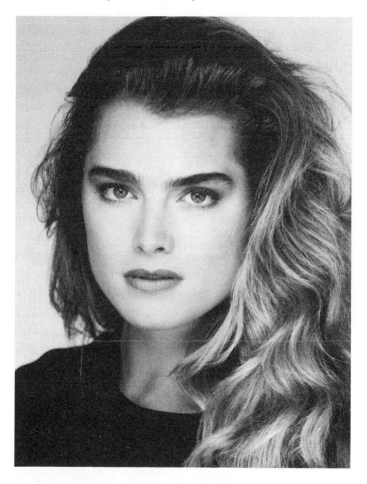

## SEXY
### As Seen On: Marilyn Monroe

Voluptuous and ultra-feminine, these sharp, sex-kitten arches ushered in a new eyebrow era in Hollywood, a welcome contrast to the skinny, swooping brows of earlier starlets. They are also a great example of how striking a dark brow can look with blond hair. Try these "come hither" arches on your next hot date. They're the brow equivalent of bedroom eyes.

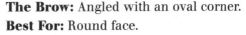 **The Brow:** Angled with an oval corner.
**Best For:** Round face.

**How to Get It: 1.** Using a brow pencil, place a visible dot right at the top point of your brow peak (this will help accentuate the angle). Then place a light dot at the inner corner of your brow and again at the end of the tail. **2.** Starting at the inner corner, brush the hairs up and toward the point of the peak. Brush the tail hairs down and toward the point of the tail. **3.** Using a brow pencil and the pictures as a guide, create an oval shape at the inner corner. **4.** Draw a straight line along the top edge from the inner corner to the dot on at your peak. Repeat with other brow. **5.** Draw a parallel line along the bottom edge of the brow. **6.** Now draw a straight line from the dot on the top of your peak to the one at the end of your tail. This creates the effect of "moving" your arch out beyond the iris—without a bit of plucking! Fill in the tail area and any blank spots with pencil or powder. Note that the tail of this brow is wider and more pronounced than the inner corner, so thicken the tail a bit, if necessary. **7.** To create a smooth edge, outline the whole brow lightly in pencil and gel in place, if necessary. Repeat with other brow.

You can also use stencil inspired by Marilyn Monroe's brow (see Resources).

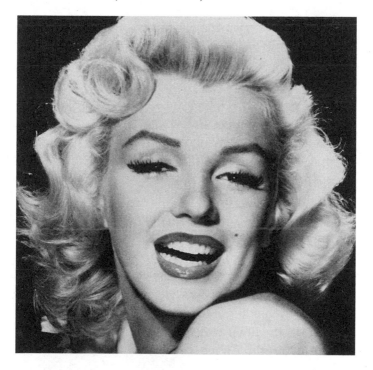

## MYSTERIOUS
### As Seen On: Diana Ross

The high, sharp arches of this brow give the face an "I know something you don't know" look that's intriguing and super sexy. This shape also lifts the whole eye area, making it seem much larger, especially when counterbalanced with smoky eyeliner smudged along the lower lids.

**The Brow:** Angled with a sleek inner corner.

**Best For:** Square or round face, or someone with almond-shaped eyes.

**How to Get It: 1.** Using a brow pencil, place a visible dot right at the top point of your brow peak (this will help accentuate the angle). Then place a light dot at the inner corner of your brow and again at the end of the tail. **2.** Starting at the inner corner, brush the hairs up and toward the point of the peak. Brush the tail hairs down and toward the point of the tail. **3.** Using a brow pencil and the pictures as a guide, create a slim, pointed oval shape at the inner corner. **4.** Draw a straight line along the top edge from the inner corner to the dot on at your peak. Repeat with other brow. **5.** Along the bottom edge, carefully draw a curve that starts at the inner corner and ends at the point of the tail. **6.** Now draw a straight line from the dot on the top of your peak to the one at the end of your tail. This creates the effect of "moving" your arch out beyond the iris. Fill in the tail area and any blank spots with pencil or powder. Note that the tail of this brow is wider and more pronounced than the inner corner, so thicken the tail a bit, if necessary. **7.** To create a smooth edge, outline the whole brow lightly in pencil and gel in place, if necessary. Repeat with other brow.

You can also use stencil inspired by Diana Ross's brow (see Resources).

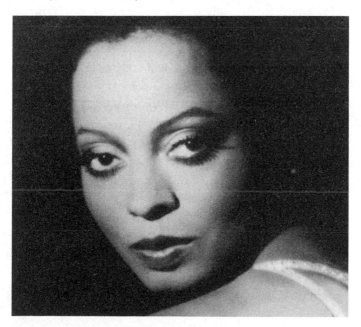

## DRAMATIC
### As Seen On: Barbra Streisand

These are eyebrows with *attitude,* perfect for when you want to play the diva. They're great at balancing strong features such as Streisand's prominent nose, and the placement of the peak just beyond the outside of the iris widens her narrow face. Even if your face is far from perfect, these brows send the message that you love the way you look. But they are not for the meek, and need to be supported by strong eye makeup. A headdress with hanging beads, however, is optional.

 **The Brow:** Angled, but with a very low arch and an oval corner.

**Best For:** Square face or someone with a prominent nose. This brow can also work for a round face if the arch is made higher.

**How to Get It: 1.** Using a brow pencil, place a visible dot right at the top point of your brow peak (this will help accentuate the angle). Then place a light dot at the inner corner of your brow and again at the end of the tail. **2.** Starting at the inner corner, brush the hairs up and toward the point of the peak. Brush the tail hairs down and toward the point of the tail. **3.** Using a brow pencil and the pictures as a guide, create an oval shape at the inner corner. **4.** Draw a straight line along the top edge from the inner corner to the dot at your peak. **5.** Draw a parallel line along the *inner half* of the bottom edge so that the bottom inner half mirrors the top. Repeat with other brow. **6.** Now draw a straight line from the dot at the top of your peak to the one at the end of your tail. This creates the effect of "moving" your arch out beyond the iris. Fill in the tail area and any blank spots with pencil or powder. **7.** To create a smooth edge, outline the whole brow lightly in pencil and gel in place, if necessary. Repeat with other brow.

You can also use stencil inspired by Barbra Streisand's brow (see Resources).

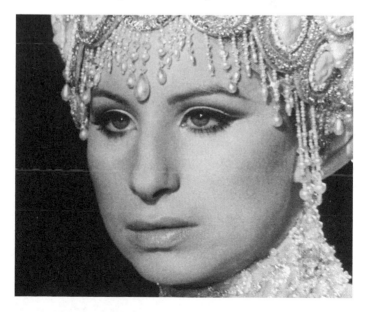

## SEDUCTIVE
## As Seen On: Sophia Loren

With their irresistible curves, these bombshell brows whisper, "I want you . . . now!" Their large size also does a darn good job of balancing Loren's large facial features without overpowering them, and the tail of the brow points down toward her strong cheekbones to ensure that you don't miss them. Caution: Wear this shape only if you're ready to really *sizzle.*

 **The Brow:** Curved with a block-shaped corner.

**Best For:** Diamond or square face, or someone with a prominent nose.

**How to Get It: 1.** Using a brow pencil, extend the inner corner of your brow straight up a bit and then carefully curve up to meet your natural peak. Create a parallel curve along the bottom edge of the brow, so that the bottom mirrors the top. Fill in any blank spots with brow powder. Repeat with other brow. **2.** Use pencil to taper the tail of your brows to a point. **3.** To create a smooth edge, outline the whole brow lightly in pencil and gel in place, if necessary. Repeat with other brow.

You can also use stencil inspired by Sophia Loren's brow (see Resources).

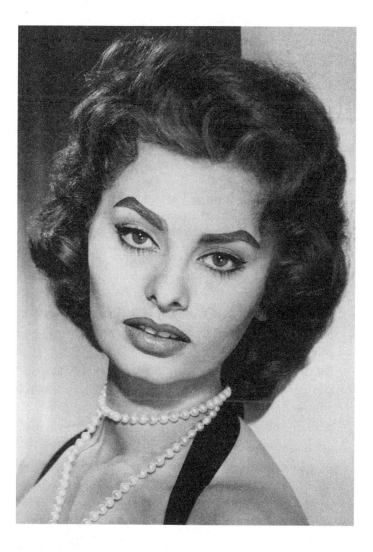

## INTELLIGENT
### As Seen On: Katharine Hepburn

These no-nonsense, straightforward brows make you look smart and confident without sacrificing your femininity. This shape also solves some common problems: The delicate thinness and gentle curves will add softness to an angular face and nicely balance a pointy chin or large lips, just the way they do for Hepburn.

**The Brow:** Rounded with a slight arch and an oval corner.

**Best For:** Slightly long face and angular features, or someone with a pointed chin or large lips.

**How to Get It: 1.** Using a brow brush, brush the hairs down and toward the outer corner. This should compress the hairs into a thinner line. Gel in place. **2.** Using a brow pencil and the pictures as a guide, carefully draw a gentle curve slightly *below* the top edge of the brow, ending at a point even with the one you started at (this will create an even thinner effect). If you feel the tail of your brow doesn't come down far enough, simply extend it lightly with pencil. **3.** To create a smooth edge, outline the whole brow lightly in pencil (following the newly defined upper edge) and gel in place, if necessary.

You can also use stencil inspired by Katharine Hepburn's brow (see Resources).

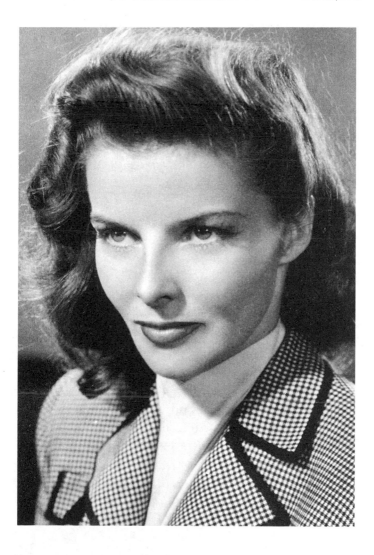

# REBELLIOUS
## As Seen On: Madonna

Like the superstar herself, this brow shape is a combination of contradictions. It starts off wild with a tufted inner corner, then turns sleek and sexy before tapering into a tail that extends way beyond the usual limits. Yet somehow it all works together to create an image of bold sexuality and strength. It's a passionate brow for a passionate woman.

**The Brow:** Rounded with a tufted teardrop corner and a very long tail.

**Best For:** Heart-shaped or very angular face, or someone with large lips.

**How to Get It: 1.** Using a brow brush, brush the hairs at the inner corner straight up to form a tuft. **2.** Brush the hairs along the top of the brow down and out toward the outer corner, and the hairs along the bottom of the brow up and toward the outer corner. This should compress the hairs into a thinner line. Gel in place. Repeat with other brow. **3.** Using a brow pencil and the pictures as a guide, create a rounded teardrop shape at the inner corner. Fill in with pencil or powder. **4.** Using pencil, draw a gentle curve along the top edge of the brow and down the tail, extending it. **5.** To create a smooth edge, outline the whole brow lightly in pencil and gel in place, if necessary. Repeat with other brow.

You can also use stencil inspired by Madonna's brow (see Resources).

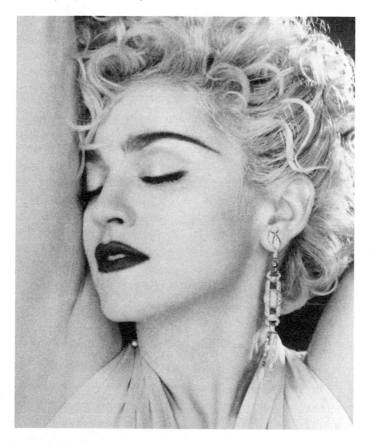

# RESOURCES

You can get great brow products and information from the following companies and organizations.

**www.eyebrowz.com.** My Web site is an on-line, one-stop resource for eyebrow information, advice, and products. See amazing brow makeovers, get step-by-step illustrated instructions for various techniques, and choose from more than one hundred eyebrow stencils inspired by celebrity shapes, as well as those based on the five basic eyebrow shapes with variations. The site also features a full line of quality eyebrow powders and pencils in a wide variety of colors, including the white pencil to help you shape your brows correctly. There's also a selection of Tweezerman tweezers, eyebrow mousses and gels, brushes and combs, even eyebrow razors. Order on-line or call 1-888-689-3389.

**International Guild of Professional Electrologists.** This organization can help you find a licensed or board-certified electrologist in your area, as well as provide more information on electrolysis for the brows and other areas. Visit www.igpe.org or call 1-800-830-3247.

**www.luxotticagroup.com.** Visit this site, run by Luxottica Eyewear, for an in-depth guide to choosing the right frame for your face shape. Click on "Selecting Eyewear" and then on "Face Shape Guide." And don't miss "Framing the Stars" to see what glasses various celebrities have worn in movies and on television shows.

**Sephora.** This makeup mega-store carries dozens of shades of mascara, perfect for coloring brows temporarily. The Sephora collection features a wide range of blacks, brows, reds, yellows, and even gray. At only a few dollars each, it's a cheap way to experiment with different brow colors. Visit a Sephora location (call 1-877-9-SEPHORA to find one near you) or order on-line at www.sephora.com.

**Tweezerman.** These tweezers are the cream of the plucking crop. The precisely ground tips are made to grab even fine hairs easily. So though they are a bit more expensive than most drugstore brands, they're worth it. And Tweezerman offers a lifetime guarantee. Visit www.tweezerman.com to see the whole line of products. You can order on-line or call 1-800-645-3340 to find a store near you.

# ABOUT THE AUTHORS

**Nancy Parker** credits her analytical ability to her background as a chemical engineer and chartered accountant. Although these two fields are seemingly unrelated to the world of beauty, it's surprising how closely aligned they actually are. All three make extensive use of the analysis of information, the sensing of patterns or trends in that information, and, most important, the development of practical tools and techniques to solve individual problems. After designing a solution to her own eyebrow issues, she began to appreciate both the role eyebrows played in individual beauty and how misunderstood this was. With her husband, she founded Eyebrowz Designs Inc. in 1997. Their rapidly growing company has successfully provided eyebrow solutions for women from around the world. The company's Web site, www.eyebrowz.com, offers women an ever increasing variety of eyebrow products, including more than one hundred eyebrow stencil shapes, brow powders, brow pencils, brow gels, tweezers, and personalized models. In addition to being a chartered accountant, Nancy holds two degrees from Queen's University.

~

Former editor-in-chief of *Woman's Day Beauty,* senior editor at *Cosmopolitan,* and articles editor at *Child,* **Nancy Kalish** is a frequent contributor to many major magazines, including *Redbook, Reader's Digest, Cosmopolitan, Fitness, McCall's, Ladies Home Journal, Parenting, Parents,* and others both here and abroad. She specializes in covering beauty, health, sex, relationships, and parenting. She is also the author of *The Nice Girl's Guide to Sensational Sex.*